Beginner's Guide to Yoga

By: Kristi Abbott

Index

If you have never tried yoga before, and are looking to start a practice, learn about yoga or try some relaxation techniques, you will find all of the ways that yoga can improve your health and help you to feel better.

Yoga is not only a physical exercise; it is a practice of quieting the mind, relaxing the body and improving mental awakening. Each of the benefits of yoga are different for everyone, and whatever reasons you may have for beginning a yoga practice, you will find the benefits for yourself.

When you begin to practice any of the asanas, or poses, you should remember to go at your own speed, and to not push yourself. Yoga is something that you can ease into and take your time learning. Yoga is one of the best ways to center yourself, focus and relax.

Beginning a yoga practice is a great step toward your wellness journey and I hope you discover all of the many ways that yoga can help you improve your life and feel better.

Tips to Get Started

1. You can do any or all of the poses in the sequence and modify the poses to fit your body
2. Choose a quiet place for your practice and you may want to listen to the audio files that accompany the book, or some relaxing or meditation music.
3. Go at your own pace. Yoga is not a way to compare yourself to others; it is a practice of listening to your body and learning to go at your own pace.
4. Practice on a good yoga mat that will help provide you with the stability and support that you need for your practice.
5. You may want to practice in bare feet if that is comfortable for you.
6. Some of the props that you may feel help you include a yoga strap, block or bolster
7. As you work through each of the poses, take your time to be present in the pose, and aware of your body and your mind
8. You may want to begin and end each of your sessions with a few minutes of meditation
9. Drink plenty of water and try not to eat or drink right before a yoga session. Try to give your body time to process each meal before movement.
10. Believe in yourself and your wellness.

Disclaimer: Before you begin any exercise program, you should first consult with your doctor to see if you are well enough to do the Yoga practice. BodySava is not responsible for any injuries or problems associated with the practice.

What is Yoga?

Basics of Hatha Yoga

There are methods of Hatha yoga that are practiced and that are known by different names. As we move through life, our bodies and minds change, therefore our yoga practice can also adapt to those changes. When beginning a yoga practice, it is important to keep the mind and heart open to receive and learn the practice.

Types of Hatha yoga:

- Viniyoga

- Iyengar

- Sivanyanda

- Bikram

- Astanga Vinyasa

Eight Limbs of yoga:

- Yama – these are the rules and restraints of conduct

- Niyama – this is the discipline of the body and the mind

- Asana – these are the steady postures that build strength, endurance and balance

- Pranayama – this is a breathing technique that is said to control the vital energy

- Pratyahara – this is preparation for meditation

- Dharana – this is the concentration and mind focus

- Dhyana – this is the meditation and ability to focus on one object

- Samadhi – this is the information and enlightenment that we take from mediation and where we recognize the true nature.

Yoga Breathing:

The ancient yogis believed that the way that we breathe is an essential component to the quality of life that we can have. Stress and anxiety are two of the factors that people face and these can be eased with proper breathing. When you learn to breathe deeply from the belly, the breath is deep and can make it easier to relax. When you practice yoga, try concentrating on focusing on the belly where the breath begins.

Benefits of Proper Breathing:

- Relaxed muscles

- Circulation of oxygenated blood

- Keeps the body healthy

- Creates heat within the body to make is more flexible and pliable

Breathing Meditation

The Breath can be a focal point in mediation. In meditation, the mind is clear and clarity can help create a new perspective on life.

History of Yoga

Yoga originated about 5000 years ago from India and was adopted by many cultures over the years. In the 1920s archeologists began discovering signs of cultures who practiced yoga when the Hindu yoga masters, or Swamis, began traveling into the west to teach yoga. In 1918, the oldest Indian technical institute of Yoga as opened in Santa Cruz, Mumbai.

Preclassical yoga began 2000 years ago until the second century. This is when the Bhagavad Gita was written and is one of the most notable yoga texts. Classical Yoga is the period of Raja yoga, which was taught by Pantanjali in his Yoga Sutra.

Postclassical yoga is the period where all of the different schools of yoga arose after Pantanjali. Hatha yoga was also conceived during this period. Modern yoga arrived in the United States in the late 1800's and became more widespread during the 1960's. Yoga has now evolved and continues to spread into many cultures and in the western culture.

Benefits of Yoga

- Improved flexibility

- Awareness of Mind and Body

- Increased strength

- Increased sense of balance

- Cleansing of the internal systems

- Enhancement of the digestive system

- Improved breathing

- Reduced anxiety

- Recovery from disease and addiction

- Personal path of discovery

- Relieves mental tension

Components of Yoga

There are nine main components of yoga.

- Asana – the body postures that cleanse and tone
- Drishti – the 9 gaze points to obtain concentration
- Suryara Maskuara – the sun salutations that consist of 12 positions
- Pranayama – the control of the vital energy through breathing. Prana means cosmic energy and the life force.
- Ujjayi – the deep thoracic breathing from the ribs that move from the back of the throat down to the heart and the rest of the body
- Bandhas – these are the energy support locks that hold the energy that is used to direct and awaken creative energy.
- Relaxation – the poses that remove anxieties and mental anguish as well as allow the body to restore itself.
- Meditation – the concentration on a particular item or object

Types of Yoga

There are over 100 types of yoga. These are some of the more popular forms of yoga that are practiced in the west.

Hatha – the discipline of the asanas, pranayama and breath control. Ha means sun, and Tha means moon.

Raja – called royal because it uses exercise and breathing practices with mediation and study.

Jnana – exercise of wisdom and knowledge

Bhatki – practice of extreme love and devotion

Karma – discipline of self surpassing action

Mantra – practice of numinous sounds that protect the mind

Laya – features that absorb the elements

Tantra – way of seeing the seen consciousness in form of thoughts, words, diagrams and movements.

Mental and Physical

Benefits of Yoga

Yoga creates a sense of accomplishment. It makes you feel like you have truly completed something good and healthy for yourself. The older we get, the more we tend to get into old habits and not try new things.

New activities like yoga bring a new and welcome change to taking charge of our health. The benefits of yoga go beyond the physical effects, and create a mental experience that can greatly improve mental health and wellness.

Some of the most notable mental benefits of yoga include:

- Clarity

- Alertness

- Achievement

- Positive Feedback

- Awakening

- Happiness

- Success

Along with the sense of accomplishment that comes with yoga, there is also a time and reason to feel good about taking care of yourself.

By learning to listen to your body, you are able to know

your limitations and abilities, and also respect what you can and cannot do. Yoga is not about comparing yourself to anyone else, or trying to do what someone else can do. It is about taking time for yourself and improving your health.

Taking the time to have a regular yoga practice may seem difficult at first, but even if you can try and set aside a few minutes a day to practice some of the asanas, or poses, and breathing techniques you will be able to see improvement.

You may find that you are able to experience benefits of yoga even when you are not practicing. Many people find that they use better posture, focus on deep breathing and feel more relaxed when they would normally be tense.

You also want to be patient with yourself. Yoga does not transform your body overnight, and you need to let your body adapt to each concept of yoga including the poses, breathing and meditation. You may not be able to do as much as you want, or be as flexible as you want at first, but if you stick with it and practice you will be able to get better and feel better.

The mental and physical benefits of yoga are often experienced at the same time because as you are learning to stretch tight muscles in the body, you are learning to expand the mind and find new ways to relax.

Physical benefits of yoga are also an important factor. It is a safe and effective way to exercise and stay fit, while learning to listen to your body and improve your health.

Some of the physical benefits of yoga include:

- Increased range of motion

- Increase in flexibility

- Easy on the joints

- Physical exercise that is gentle

- Strength building

- Balance

- Relief from chronic fatigue or pain

- Slow down symptoms of chronic illness

- Improved coordination and circulation

Beginner's Yoga Routine

This yoga sequence is designed to provide an easy and gentle practice. The poses, or asanas, are gentle and basic and can be modified to accommodate physical limitations.

Each of the poses in the sequence can be performed on its own or as part of the sequence. The important thing to remember when beginning a yoga practice is to listen to your body. Your body will let you know when you have pushed too far, or when you need to ease up. Learning to be in tune with your body is one of the main benefits of a yoga practice.

The illustrations show how the pose is performed, and the descriptions show how you can modify each of the poses to make it more comfortable and easy to perform.

Simple Crossed Legged Pose

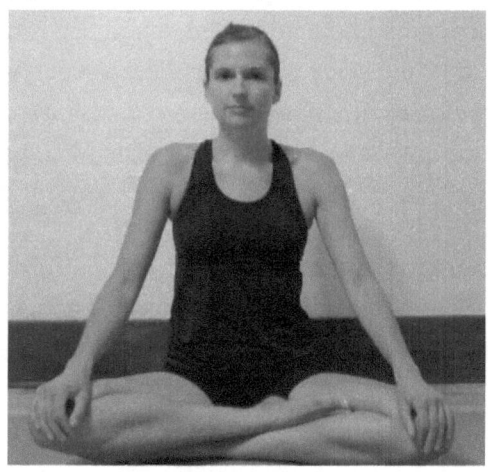

This pose can be performed as shown or you can relax the legs out in front if that is more comfortable for the knees.

Posture: **Begin in simple cross legged pose. You can cross the legs and either have the feet on the thighs, or on the floor. Let your hands rest lightly on the knees with the palms up. Keep the back straight and chest open.**

Focus of Pose: **Begin to focus on your breathing. Feel the breath start deep in the belly and up through the chest, and out the nose. Feel the breath come back in through the nose, and empty into the belly. Keep the sitting bones grounded into the mat.**

Length of Pose: **10-12 breaths**

Benefits of pose: **Begin to focus on the breath and quiet the busy mind. This pose is a great way to work into your practice and become aware of yourself and your surroundings.**

Tips and Modifications: **If it is uncomfortable for you to sit with your legs crossed, you may stretch them out along the ground and bend the knees slightly. Try to keep the shoulders back and the chest open to allow for complete flow of breath.**

Happy Twist

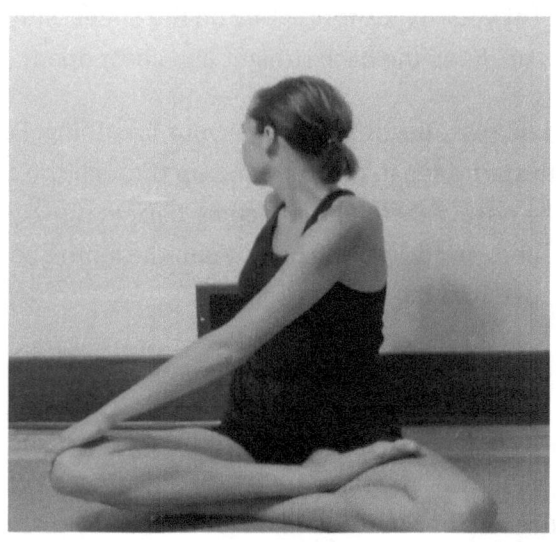

Posture: Begin in a simple crossed legged pose. Keep the spine long and the chest open. Place both hands gently on the knees. Take a breath in and open the chest completely. Exhale and slowly twist to the side bringing your left hand to the right knee and the right hand behind you. Deepen the stretch and gaze softly over the right shoulder. Hold for 10-12 breaths and slowly return to center. Repeat on the other side taking the right hand to the left knee and the left hand behind you, gazing softly over the left shoulder.

Focus of Pose: Stretch the entire spine throughout the pose and twist further on each exhale during the twist.

Length of Pose: 10-12 breaths

Benefits of pose: This is a gentle stretch for the entire spine and muscles around the spine. It is also a good way to gain range of motion.

Tips and Modifications: Try to deepen the twist and stretch on each exhale during the phase. Be sure to take even breaths and let your body adjust naturally to each move.

Cat and Cow Pose

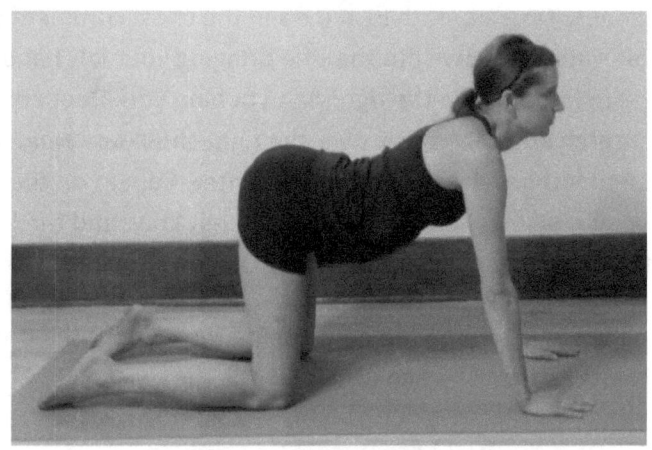

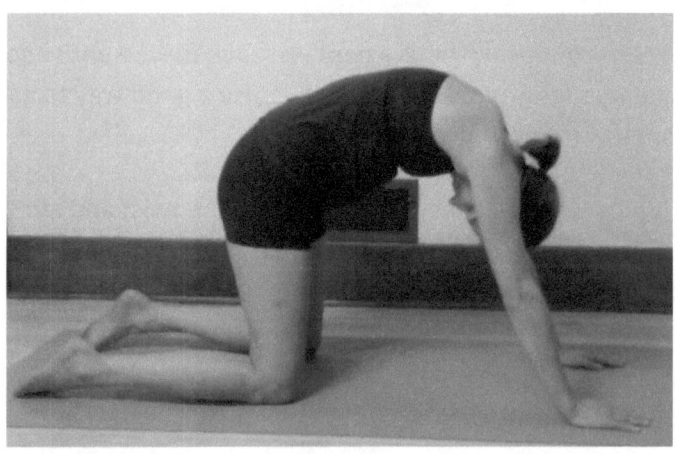

Posture: **Begin on the hands and knees. Try to keep the knees and the hands about shoulder width apart. Keep the hands even and the knees balanced. Inhale and let the belly dip towards the floor as you raise the chin up towards the sky. Exhale and let the back arch and tuck the chin in towards the chest. Hold each segment of the pose for a couple of breaths and repeat the sequence two or three times.**

Focus of Pose: **Arching the back allows the spine to warm up and to stretch. Each time that you enhance the strength of the spine, you are gaining strength in the core muscles around the back.**

Length of Pose: **10-12 breaths**

Benefits of pose: **Strengthen the back and neck muscles. Creating a subtle spine that is more flexible and strong.**

Tips and Modifications: **Try to let the back arch up and feel each vertebrae as they are stretching during the cat phase of the pose, and feel each vertebrae relax and become subtle during the cow phase of the pose.**

Arm and Leg Extension

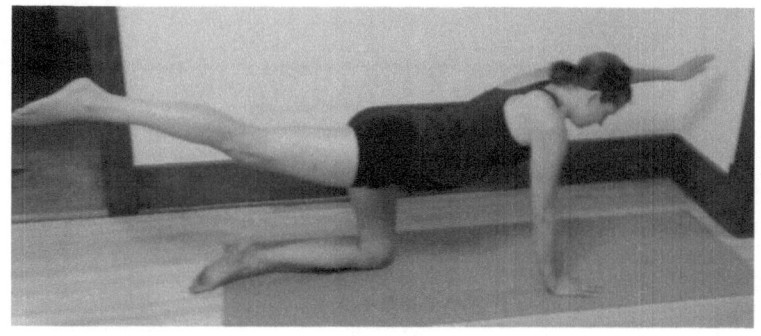

Posture: **Begin on the hands and knees. Take a deep breath in and exhale. On the next deep breath in raise up the left arm and extend it out in front of you. Try to reach out from the shoulder through the finger tips and let the eyes gaze softly towards the mat. Lower the arm back down and repeat with the right arm. With both hands on the floor, inhale and lift the left leg up and extend it behind you. Hold and lower the leg back down, bringing the right leg up and out behind you.**

Focus of Pose: **Balance the entire body by learning how to shift the weight of your body from each arm when extended, and from each leg when extended.**

Length of Pose: **10-12 breaths**

Benefits of pose: **Building strength throughout the core muscles and the arms and legs. Balancing of the body by learning to shift weight between the arms and the legs and maintain a strong base.**

Tips and Modifications: **When you are extending the arms during the pose, try to reach out from the shoulder to the finger tips. When you are extending the legs, try to keep the hips balanced.**

Child's Pose

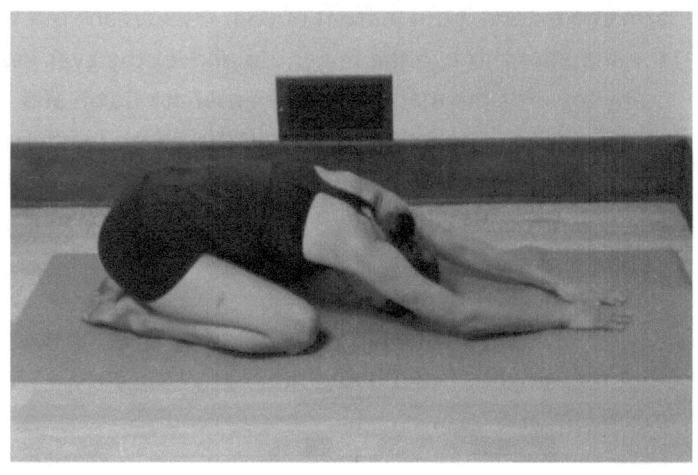

Posture: **Lean back on the ankles and extend the arms out in front of you. Lower the head towards the mat. Relax into the pose as you deepen the stretch. Each time that you exhale, try to walk the fingers out a little further in front of you.**

Focus of Pose: **Relaxing the body while stretching out the arms and the hips after extensions.**

Length of Pose: **10-12 breaths**

Benefits of pose: **Stretching out the muscles after extensions, and allowing the body to rest while stretching and warming the hips and shoulders.**

Tips and Modifications: **If it is not uncomfortable for you to lean forward on the floor or lower your head to the floor, take a folded chair in front of you and lower down only to the level of the chair, resting your arms and head on the seat.**

Gate Pose

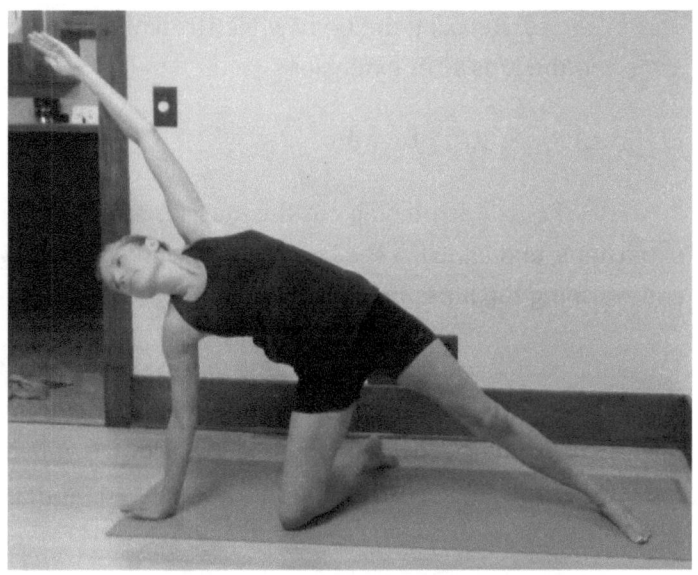

Posture: **Begin on both knees. Inhale and step the left foot out to the side. Exhale and bring the right arm up and over the head as you bring the left hand down on the knee or top of the left leg. Hold and deepen the stretch. Slowly inhale and come back to center and repeat to the right side.**

Focus of Pose: **This pose opens the rib cage and chest and also allows you to strengthen the muscles of the leg. Try to reach up with the opposite hand overhead as you press down and away from the opposite knee during each side of the stretch.**

Length of Pose: **10-12 breaths**

Benefits of pose: **Opens the chest and rib cage. Opens and stretches the hip and outer thigh muscles. Strengthens the muscles of the legs.**

Tips and Modifications: **You can either look up at the opposite hand during each side of the pose, or if it is putting strain on your neck, turn and look down at the opposite leg or gaze softly in front.**

Standing Forward Bend

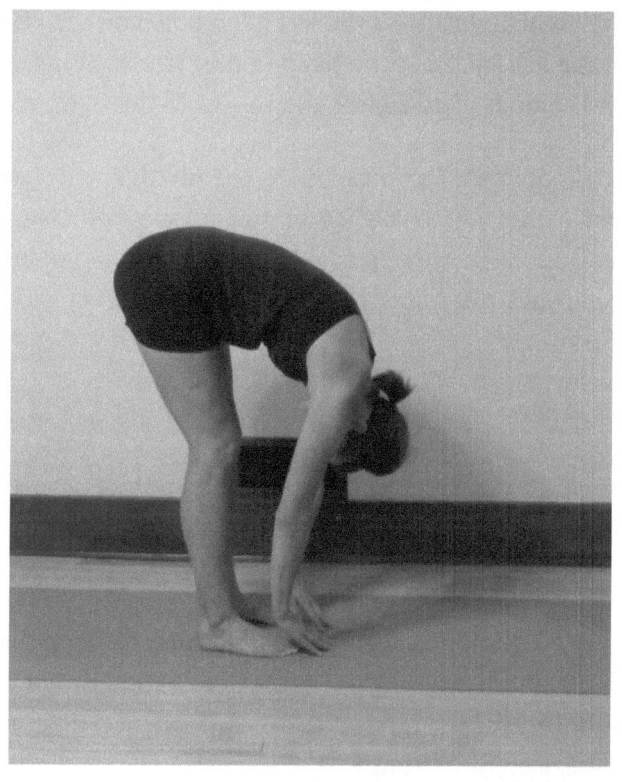

Posture: Stand with the feet together or shoulder width apart. You can either keep the knees bent or straight. Try to release the weight of the upper body, shoulders and head while you are in the pose and you can either look forward to take pressure off of your neck, or gaze softly towards the ground at your feet.

Focus of Pose: Stretch the entire spine and back of the legs. Try to let yourself go deeper into the stretch and further on each exhale and focus on stretching the entire length of the spine.

Length of Pose: 10-12 breaths

Benefits of pose: Stretches and opens the back muscles and the back of the legs. Strengthens the legs and adds flexibility to the entire body.

Tips and Modifications: If you feel uncomfortable keeping the legs straight during the pose, bend the knees softly and take pressure off of the spine.

Mountain Pose

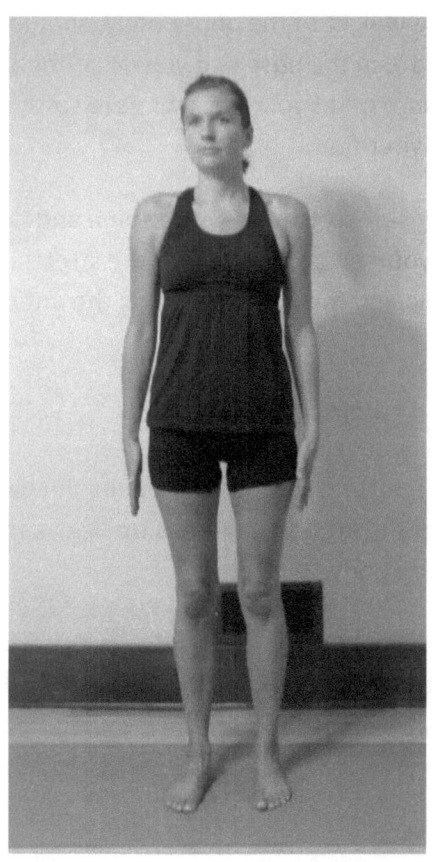

Posture: Stand with the feet about shoulder width apart. Keep the back straight and the shoulders back. Keep the chest open and stand with the arms at the sides with the fingers spread open and toes spread on the ground. Let the eyes gaze forward.

Focus of Pose: Keep the shoulders back during the pose to help open up the chest and allow for proper breathing. The strength of the legs supports the body and allows for proper stance and posture for the spine and ribcage.

Length of Pose: 10-12 breaths

Benefits of pose: Develop proper stance and balance in the body. Teach the body to align naturally and allows the spine to elongate and the chest be open to properly breathe.

Tips and Modifications: It may seem difficult at first to grasp the complexity of this pose, but try to focus on something different each time that you can improve on, such as keeping the hands still at the sides, or the toes spread openly on the floor.

Eagle

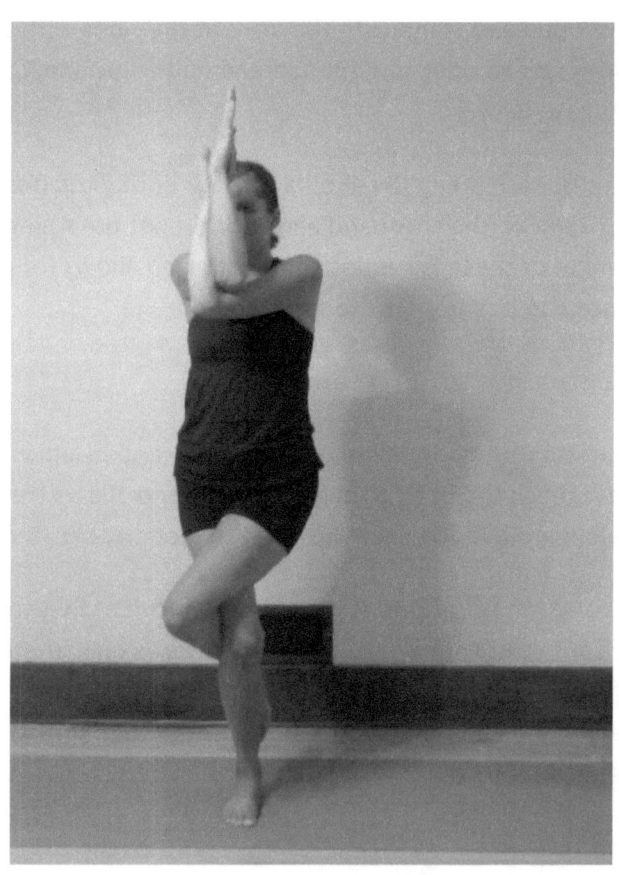

Posture: Begin in mountain pose. Inhale and bring both arms overhead. Exhale and bring both arms down the center together. Cross the left arm over the right arm at the elbow and bring the hands together.

Focus of Pose: Keep the shoulders as loose and low as possible to allow yourself to gain the flexibility that you need to cross the arms and hands. As you gain balance, you are able to hold the pose longer and deepen the pose through the knees as you cross the legs.

Length of Pose: **10-12 breaths**

Benefits of pose: Creates more flexibility in the shoulders which allows you to get deeper into the stretch and also builds strength in the legs as you begin to gain more balance.

Tips and Modifications: If it is not easy for you to cross your hands during the pose, bring them as close together as you can. You can bend the knees and stop at the point instead of crossing the legs if it is difficult to balance in the pose. As you shoulders loosen up and you gain more flexibility, you are able to get further into the pose and cross the arms and hands easier.

Wrist Stretch

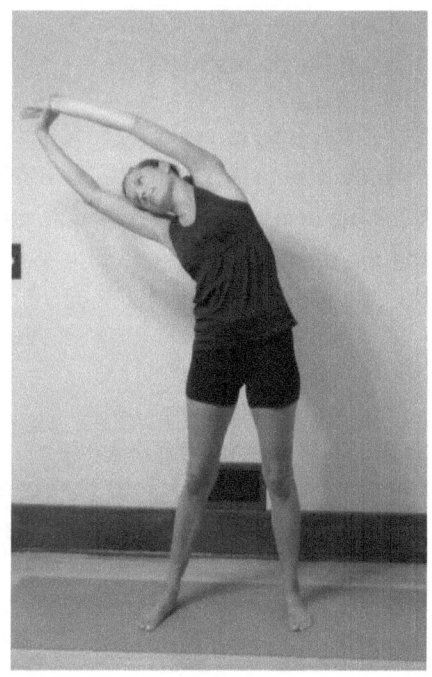

Posture: Begin in mountain pose or in a crossed legged position if you are on the floor. Inhale and bring both arms overhead. Exhale and take the left wrist in the right hand, stretching down to the right. Hold and release both arms. Inhale and bring the arms overhead, exhale and take the right wrist in the left hand and stretch down to the left.

Focus of Pose: Open up the entire side and ribcage. Open up the hips and focus on the flexibility that you gain each time you stretch during the pose.

Length of Pose: 10-12 breaths

Benefits of pose: Create more flexibility in the hips, shoulders and builds strength through the upper body and back.

Tips and Modifications: Only go as far into the stretch as you feel comfortable. You can always work on gaining more flexibility as you continue your practice. It is more important to ease into each stretch during the pose and not go as deep as you would like at first.

Tree

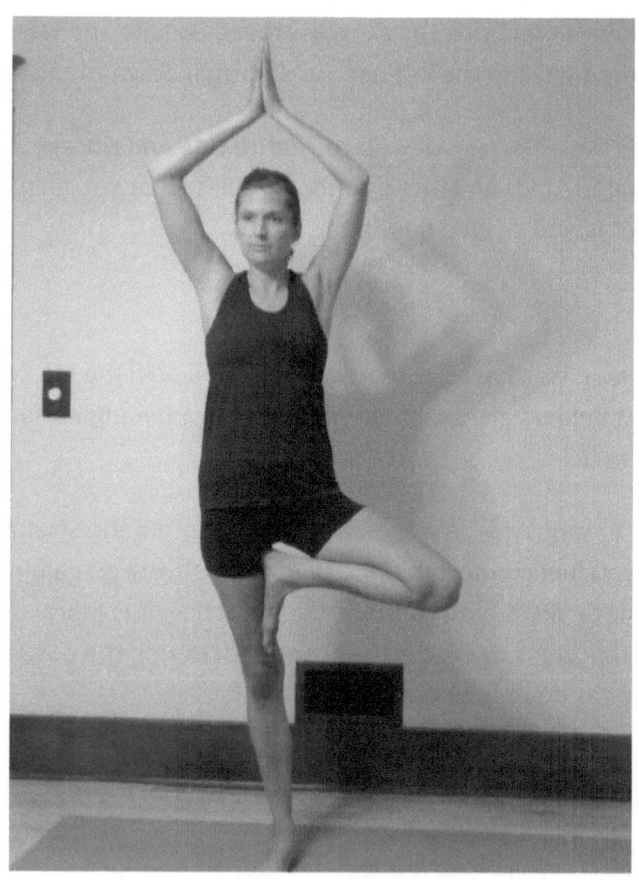

Posture: **Begin in mountain pose. Take the left heel and place it against the right leg. Inhale and bring both arms overhead or out to the sides to help balance. You can either keep the heel against the leg, or to move into full tree pose bring the foot up onto the right leg. Hold and repeat on the other side.**

Focus of Pose: **Use the breath to help balance in the pose. Find a place to softly gaze ahead of you to help focus on the breathing and balance during the pose.**

Length of Pose: **10-12 breaths**

Benefits of pose: **Teaches the body to balance itself and to build strength by using many muscle groups to help create the balance.**

Tips and Modifications: **If you are more comfortable beginning the pose by keeping the heel against the leg and still touching the floor, you can hold on to the wall or a chair with the other arm until you feel balanced. Try to keep the hips open and forward during the pose.**

Sobriety Focus: **Balance is difficult to maintain when you are beginning sobriety, but the more that you practice and the more that you believe that you can do it, you will be able to.**

Wide Legged Forward Bend

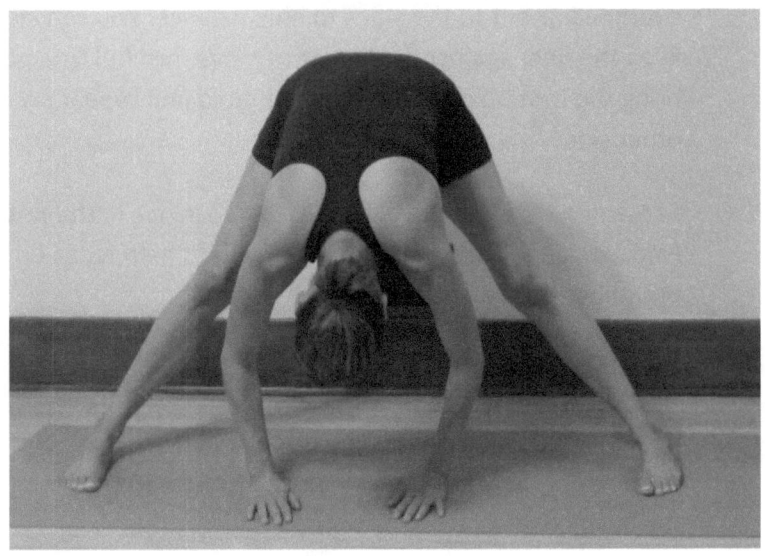

Posture: Begin in mountain pose. Spread the legs a little wider than shoulder width apart. Inhale and bring both arms overhead. Exhale and lower the arms halfway. Bend from the hips down into a wide forward bend.

Focus of Pose: Bending from the hips allows you to stretch the back muscles and the back of the legs during the stretch. Try to keep focused on going a little deeper into the stretch on each exhale.

Length of Pose: **10-12 breaths**

Benefits of pose: Stretches the legs, hips and back. Builds strength from the core muscles and helps to elongate the spine.

Tips and Modifications: If it is uncomfortable for you to bring the hands towards the floor, or if you feel any pressure in the back or neck, bend the knees and rest the elbows on the legs.

Warrior II

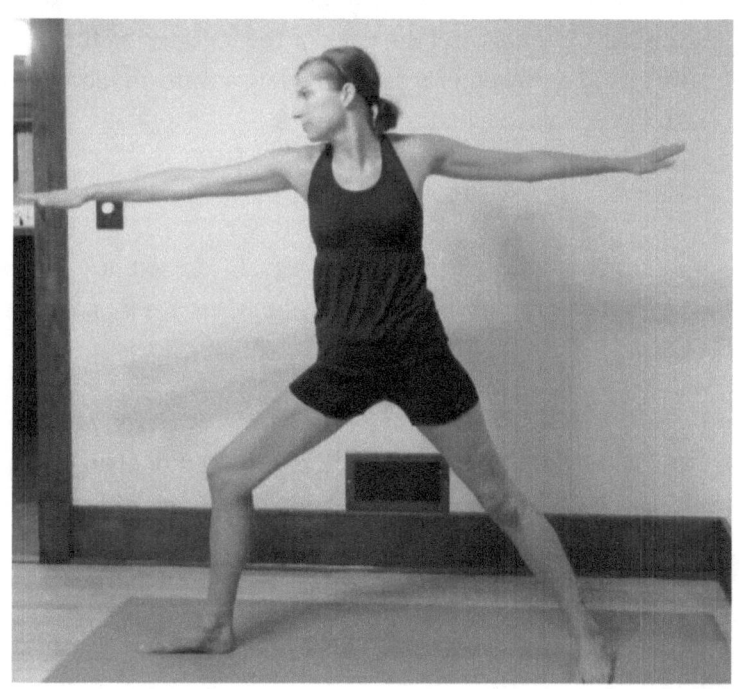

Posture: **Begin in mountain pose. Step the feet wider than shoulder width apart. Turn the right toes out to the side, and the left toes forward. Inhale and bring both arms overhead. Exhale and lower the arms halfway. Inhale and bend the right knee and look over the right shoulder. Hold and repeat on the other side.**

Focus of Pose: **Imagine that there is a line that connects the left hand and the right hand. Try to keep your knee bent only as far as you can still see the toes. Reach out through both hands and hold the body strong while you keep the chest open and the back strong.**

Length of Pose: **10-12 breaths**

Benefits of pose: **Opens up the hips and the chest. Strengthens the legs and the arms while creating balance in the body.**

Tips and Modifications: **Try to reach out towards the wall with both hands and push up from the feet to help keep the arms level and the back straight and balanced.**

Triangle Pose

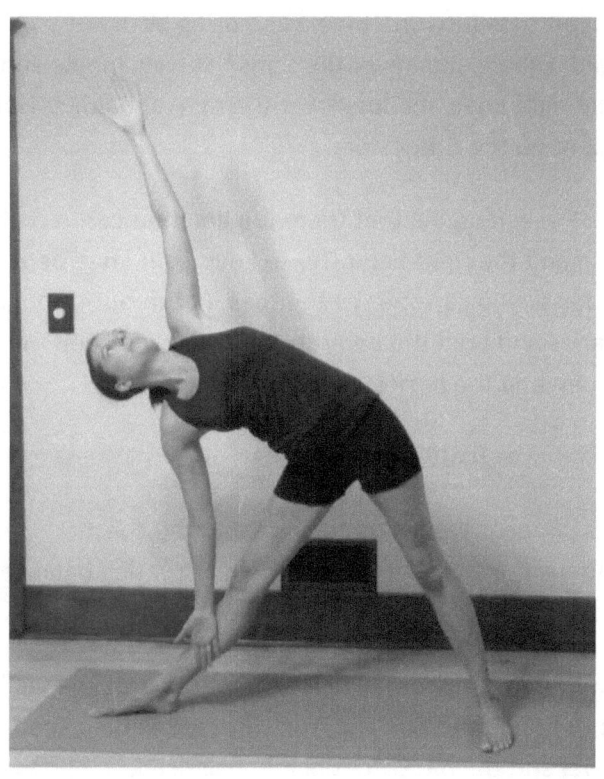

Posture: Begin in Mountain pose. Keep the feet a little wider than shoulder width apart. Turn the left toes forward and the right toes out to the side. Inhale and bring both arms overhead. Exhale and lower the arms half way. Bend from the hip and stretch down towards the right leg reaching the hand towards the ground. Raise the left arm in the air. Hold and repeat for the other side.

Focus of Pose: Open up the sides of the body and open the hips. Try to bend from the hip and stand with the hips forward.

Length of Pose: 10-12 breaths

Benefits of pose: Opens the hips and sides of the body. Strengthens the leg muscles and the arms. Stretches the side of the body and the legs.

Tips and Modifications: If it is uncomfortable for you to gaze up towards the raised hand in the pose, you may look forward or look down towards the leg.

Chair Pose

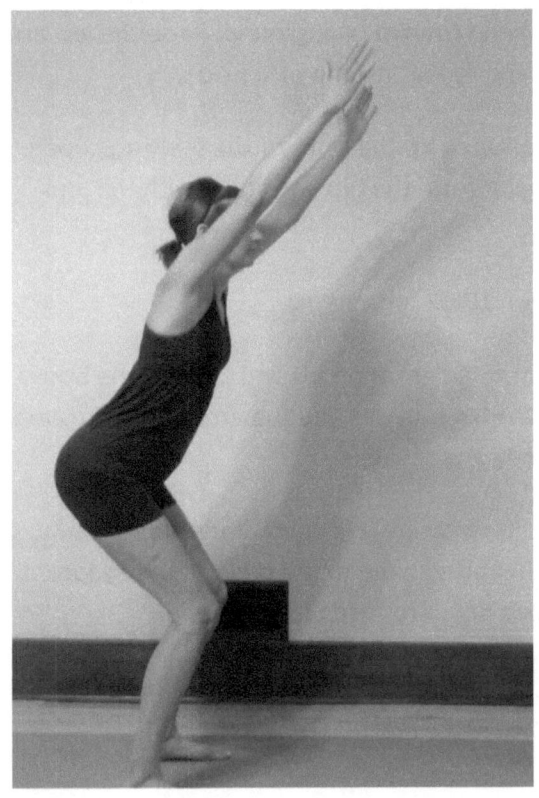

Posture: Begin in mountain pose. Step the feet about shoulder width apart. Inhale and bring both arms overhead. Exhale and keep the arms up and keep them about shoulder width apart, hands open. Bend the knees slightly and sit back like you were sitting in a chair.

Focus of Pose: Focus on keeping the arms reaching up and the legs bent slightly. Be sure that you can still see your toes and feel the stretch through the back of the legs and the back.

Length of Pose: 10-12 breaths

Benefits of pose: Stretches the back and strengthens the back, legs and arms.

Tips and Modifications: Reach up from the arms through the hands and if it is uncomfortable for you to hold the pose, take small breaks and go back into the pose.

Plank Pose

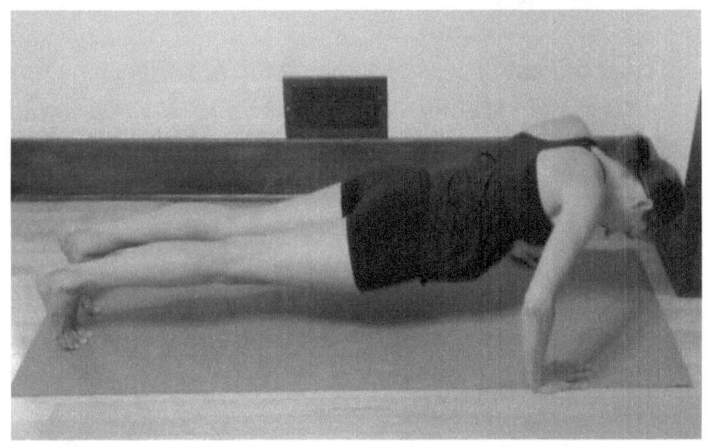

Posture: Begin with your hands on the ground and the feet touching the ground. Begin to lower yourself towards the ground and try to keep the body straight. You can bend the elbows and imagine a straight line from your entire body.

Focus of Pose: Focus on keeping the body in a line and holding yourself up from the ground. Try to hold the pose if you can, and bend the elbows to bring yourself closer to the ground.

Length of Pose: 10-12 breaths

Benefits of pose: Stretches the entire length of the spine and strengthens the arms and upper body.

Tips and Modifications: If you are not able to hold yourself up for the pose, you can bend the knees to the ground to take pressure off of the arms or back.

Upward Facing Dog

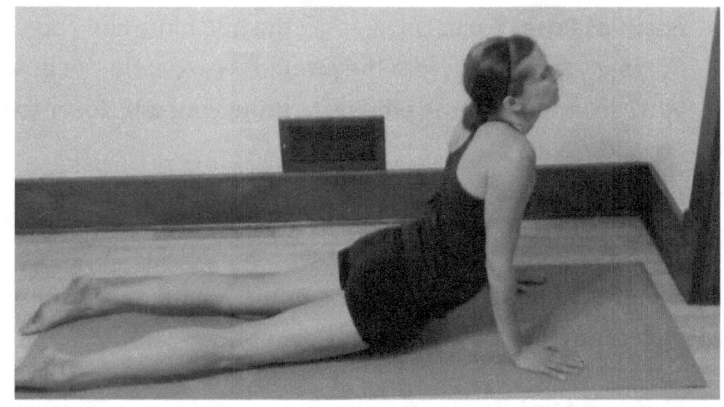

Posture: Begin by pushing yourself off of the ground from the hands. Keep the lower body and the legs touching the ground. Straighten the elbows until your upper body is elevated. You can lift the hips off of the ground.

Focus of Pose: Focus on raising the upper body off of the ground as you raise your head up and hold the arms strong to create a stronger upper body.

Length of Pose: 10-12 breaths

Benefits of pose: Stretches the arms, back and lower body while it strengthens the arms and upper body.

Tips and Modifications: If it is uncomfortable for you to lift your hips off of the ground, you can leave the hips touching the ground and raise only the upper body and arms.

Downward Facing Dog

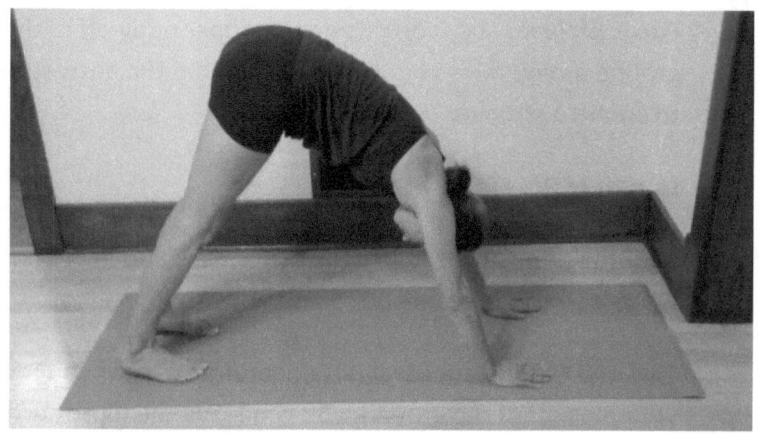

Posture: Begin by placing the hands on the ground in front of the body and the feet on the floor. You want to reach down through the heels into the ground as you push away from the ground. You can keep the legs extended or bend the knees.

Focus of Pose: Focus on pushing the weight of the body off of your hands and down the legs to the feet. Try to lower the feet to the floor, and use each exhale to deepen the stretch and press down through the heels.

Length of Pose: 10-12 breaths

Benefits of pose: Stretches the back of the body and strengthens the legs and the arms. Adds flexibility to the legs and the muscles in the back.

Tips and Modifications: If it is uncomfortable for you to hold the pose, you may bend the knees and lower the knees to the floor.

Side Plank Pose

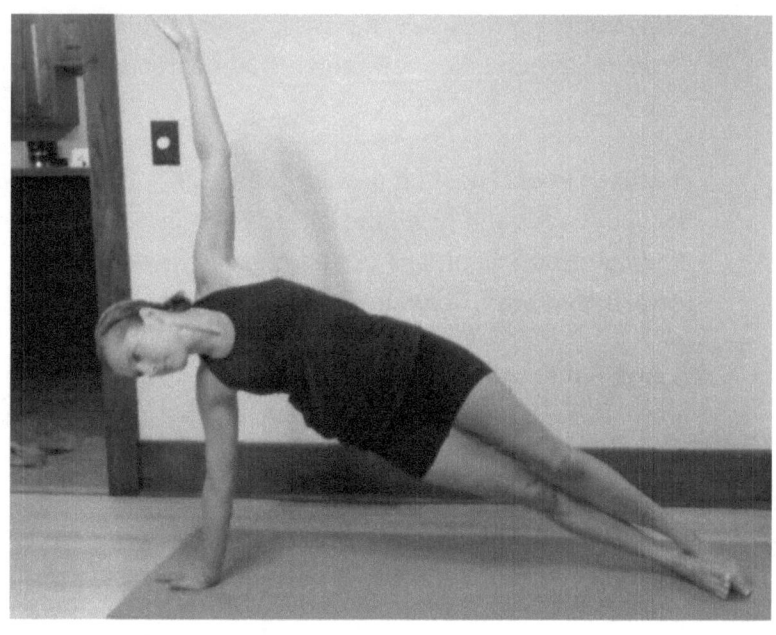

Posture: Begin on your left side. Place the left elbow on the ground and the right hand in front of you on the ground. Inhale and lift the body up, supporting yourself on the elbow and extend the right arm up in the air. You can stay in that modification, or you can lift up to the left hand and extend the right leg, balancing on the feet. Hold and repeat on the other side.

Focus of Pose: Focus on keeping the body lifting up and holding the body strong and not sinking towards the ground. Lift up from the right hand and off of the feet.

Length of Pose: 10-12 breaths

Benefits of pose: Stretches the side of the body and strengthens the back, arms and legs. Builds balance by using the elbow or hand, and the feet for support.

Tips and Modifications: If you are not able to fully extend onto the left hand, you can stay with your elbow on the ground.

Boat Pose

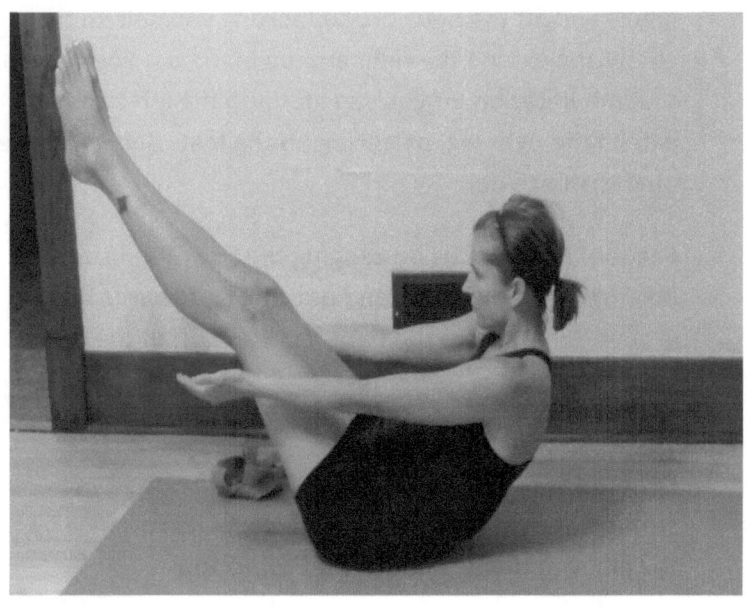

Posture: Begin with both legs extended in front of you. Bend the knees and keep the feet on the ground. Inhale and bring the hands to the thighs. Exhale and lift the feet up from the ground. You can stay with your hands on the thighs to support your back, or you can release the hands and extend the legs and arms out or up.

Focus of Pose: Focus on holding still during the pose and if you are not able to extend the arms out or the legs, try to use the abs to bring you closer to the legs.

Length of Pose: 10-12 breaths

Benefits of pose: Stretches the back and the legs. Strengthens the abs and back while building balance.

Tips and Modifications: You can stay with your hands on the legs for support and to help get used to the pose, until you are comfortable with letting the hands off of the legs and extending them out.

Camel Pose

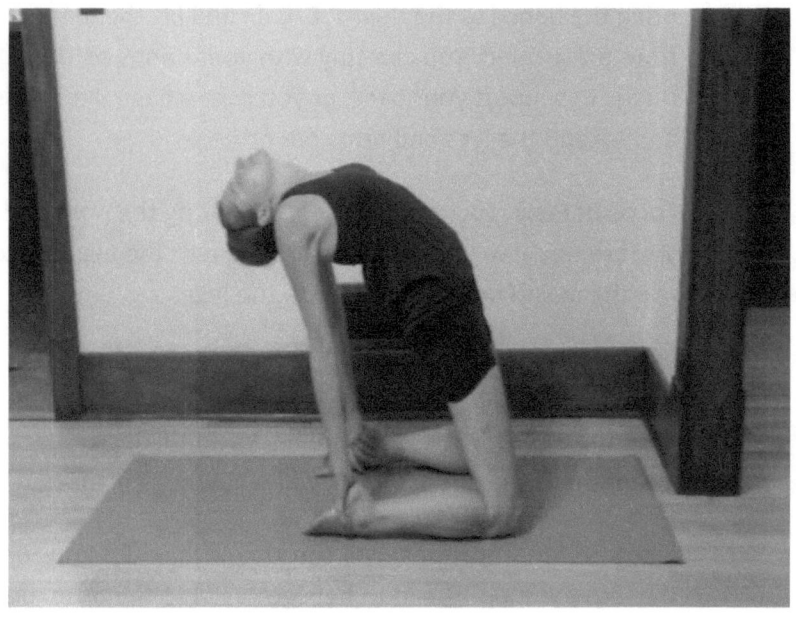

Posture: Begin on the knees. Inhale and reach the arms up. Exhale and reach the arms back, or bring them around the back to hold onto the ankles. Arch the back and stretch back towards the legs as you open up the chest. You can either stay in the position like this, or you can start by placing the hands on the lower back and working your way down towards the ankles.

Focus of Pose: Focus on keeping the chest open and the back strong as you lower down into the pose. Feel the hips open and the legs be strong.

Length of Pose: 10-12 breaths

Benefits of pose: Stretches the chest, hips and legs. Strengthens the back and the legs as you stretch the back.

Tips and Modifications: You can begin by placing the hands on the lower back on the sacrum. Lean back until you can feel a good stretch, and if you feel like you are strong, reach back down towards the ankles and hold on to the ankles.

Plow Pose

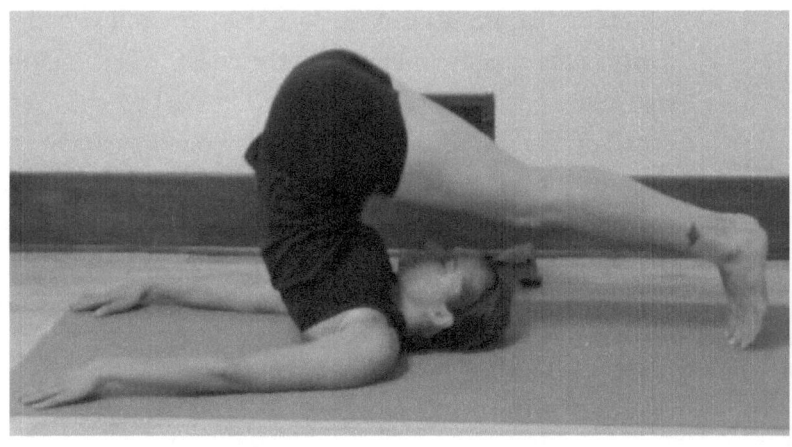

Posture: Begin on the back. Bend the knees and lift them off of the ground. Inhale and lift the legs up in the air and extend them up. Exhale and place the hands along the body on the ground, underneath of the lower back. Begin to lift up the legs and the hips, as you bring them back over the body. You can lower the legs back and over the body, bringing the feet towards the floor.

Focus of Pose : Focus on the strength of the back and the flexibility that you have in the back and legs.

Length of Pose: 10-12 breaths

Benefits of pose: Stretches the back and legs and strengthens the back.

Tips and Modifications: If you are not able to reach the legs over the head, or bring your toes to the ground behind the head, you can lift and raise the legs up and keep them in the air while you are supporting the lower back with your hands.

Crane Pose

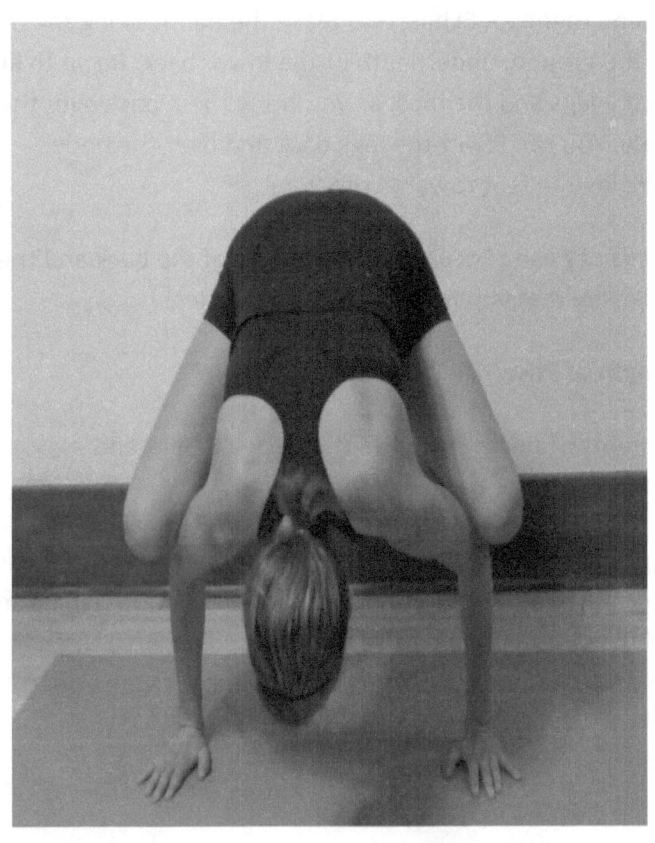

Posture: Begin with the feet on the ground and the arms in front of the legs. Let the knees rest against the arms. Begin to lean forward and lift the toes off the ground. You may need to balance for a while going forward and taking the feet off the ground until you feel stable. Once you have created balance, keep the knees on the upper arms and lift the feet up.

Focus of Pose : Focus on balancing the body and using upper body strength to support the body during the pose.

Length of Pose: 10-12 breaths

Benefits of pose: Stretches the back, strengthens the arms , opens the groin muscles and strengthens the abdominals.

Tips and Modifications: If you are not able to lift the feet off the ground and balance them on the arms, you can practice lifting one foot up at a time or stay in the position with the knees resting against the arms and hold onto the stretch.

Staff Pose

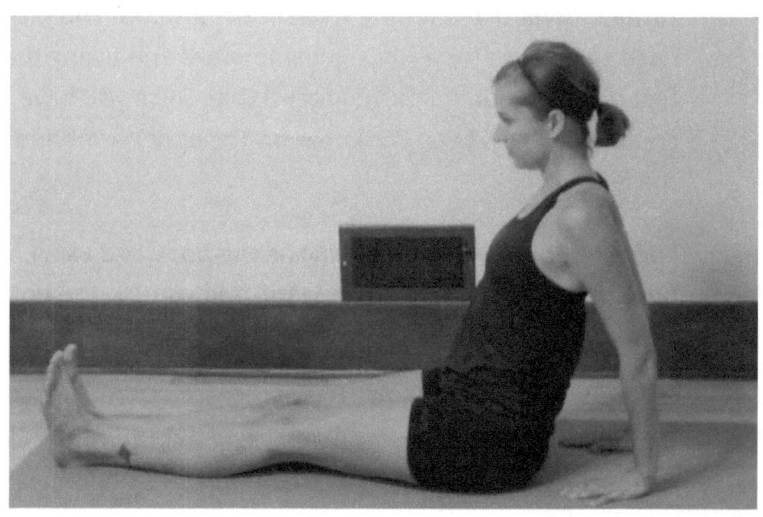

Posture: Begin with both legs extended out on the ground. Place your hands behind your body with the fingers pointed in back. Inhale and lift to open the chest and straighten the back. Exhale and deepen the stretch by opening the chest and letting the shoulders go back.

Focus of Pose: Focus on the openness that you feel in the chest and in the strength that you feel in the upper body.

Length of Pose: 10-12 breaths

Benefits of pose: Stretches the back and opens the chest. Strengthens the back muscles and the arms.

Tips and Modifications: If you are not able to hold the pose for an extended amount of time, take small breaks after each exhale and begin again in the pose.

Seated Forward Bend

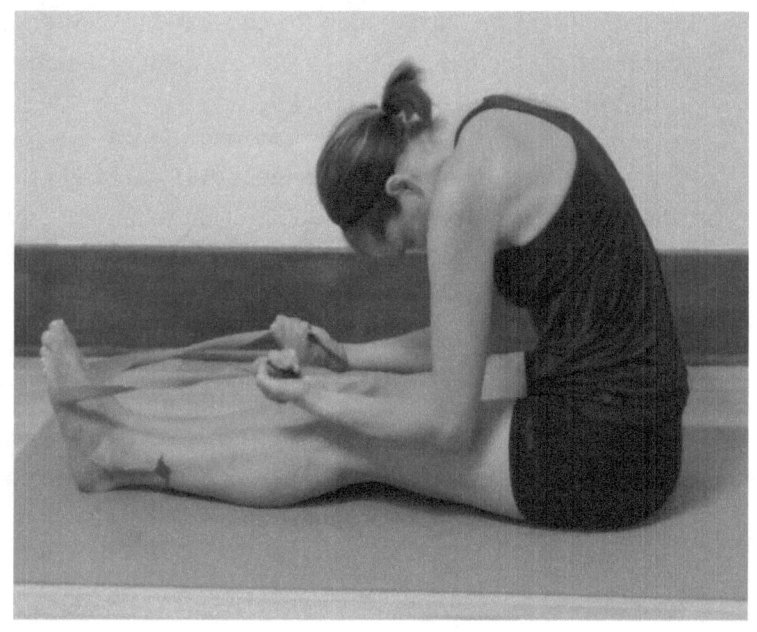

Posture: **Begin with both legs extended out in front of you. Inhale and bring the arms overhead. Exhale and lower the body down over the legs bringing your hands towards the feet.**

Focus of Pose: **Focus on going further into the stretch on each exhale and bringing the body towards the legs.**

Length of Pose: **10-12 breaths**

Benefits of pose: **Stretches the back and strengthens the lower body and the arms. Creates flexibility throughout the body and in the legs.**

Tips and Modifications: **Only go as far as you can feel a good stretch. It is ok if you are not able to reach the toes, bring your arms down as far as you can and try to go a little further on each exhale.**

Seated Forward Bend One Leg

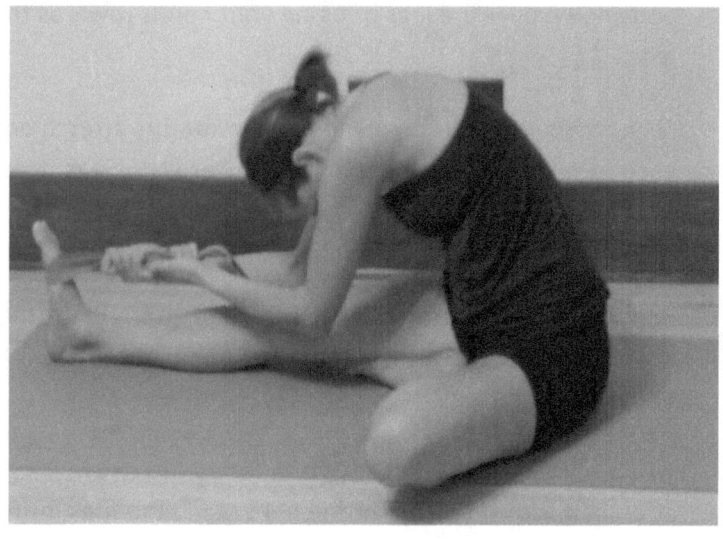

Posture: **Begin with both legs extended in front of you. Inhale and keep the right leg extended out and exhale to bend the left knee down. Inhale and bring the arms overhead. Exhale and lower both arms over the right leg. Hold and repeat to the other side.**

Focus of Pose: **Focus on stretching each leg that is extended and on stretching further towards the leg on each exhale.**

Length of Pose: **10-12 breaths**

Benefits of pose: **Stretches the leg, back and side of the body. Builds strength in the legs and the back.**

Tips and Modifications: **It is ok if you are not able to reach the toe, you can stretch down as far as you can and try to reach a little bit further on each exhale.**

Reclining Big Toe Pose

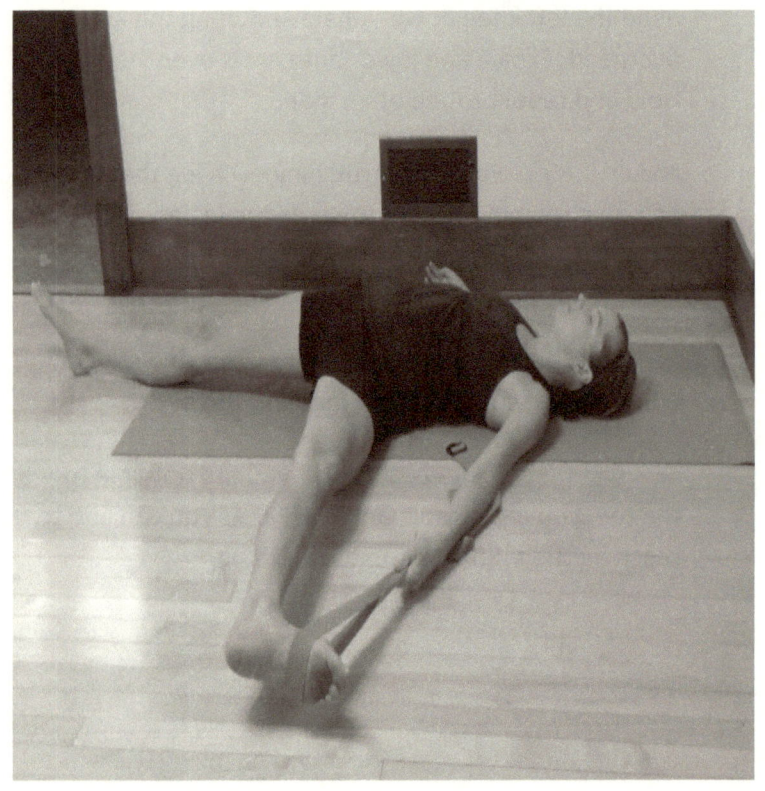

Posture: Begin on the back and extend both legs out along the ground. Keep the arms at the sides and inhale. On the exhale, bend the right knee into the chest and grab onto the big toe. Inhale, and on the exhale straighten the leg in the air. This pose can also be performed using a strap that you place around the foot. Hold and repeat on the other side.

Focus of Pose: Try to focus on extending the leg further during each exhale and using the breath to help you stretch into the pose. Feel the openness in the hips and in the legs while you are extending each leg.

Length of Pose: 10-12 breaths

Benefits of pose: This pose strengthens the back muscles and stretches out the legs and arms. This pose also opens up the hips and releases tightness in the legs and hips.

Tips and Modifications: You can use a strap to place around each foot in the pose. You can also place a blanket or bolster under the small of the back for this reclined pose to take pressure off of the spine.

Knee Hug

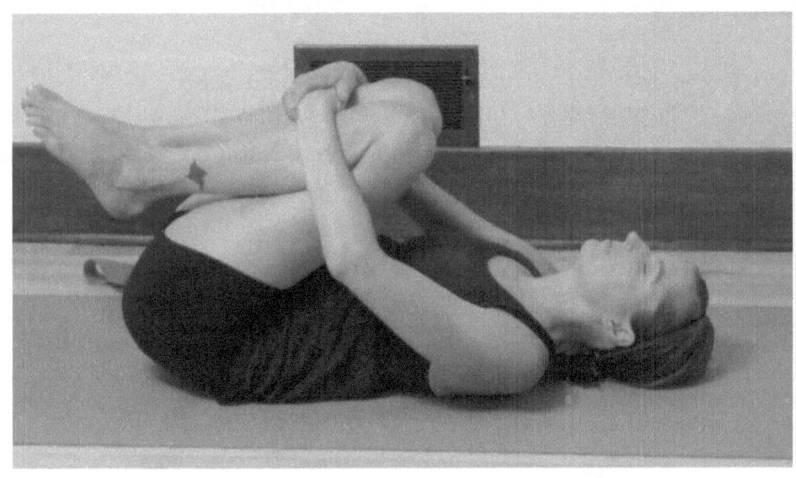

Posture: **Begin on the back. Inhale and bend both knees into the chest. Exhale and hold onto the knees with your hands and gently lift your head toward the legs. Hold and release back to the ground.**

Focus of Pose: When you are reaching up to the knees, engage the ab muscles to pull you towards the legs and feel the small of the back pressed gently into the floor. Feel the stretch in the hips and in the legs.

Length of Pose: **10-12 breaths**

Benefits of pose: This pose helps to release tension in the hips and in the legs and it also strengthens the back muscles. You can feel the muscles relaxing throughout the legs and in the hips.

Tips and Modifications: You can cross the feet during this pose to emphasize the stretch on each side of the body. You can hold the stretch with the feet crossed one way, and then cross the opposite way to stretch both sides.

Reclining Bound Ankle Pose

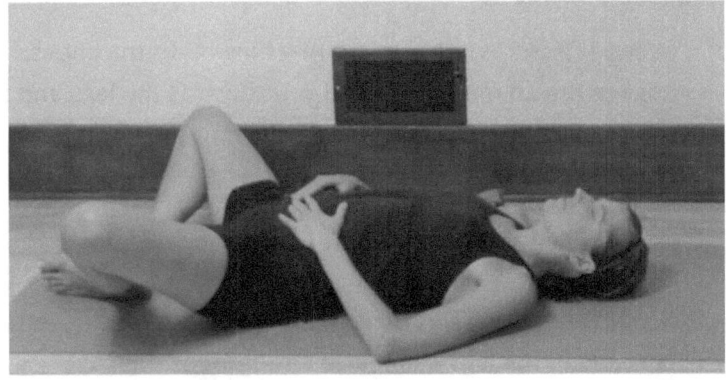

Posture: You can perform this pose lying down or sitting up. If you do the pose in this sequence, you will want to perform it on your back with the knees open and feet together. Keep the hands on the belly and relax the elbows. Inhale and feel how the belly expands, filling your hands. Exhale, and feel how the belly empties. Continue to feel the rise and fall of the belly.

Focus of Pose: This pose helps to focus on deep breathing. You want to feel the breath start deep in the belly and feel the rise and fall of each breath in your hands. Be mindful of the softness of the belly during the pose. Feel the tension in the hips and in the legs as you use each breath to relax them.

Length of Pose: 10-12 breaths

Benefits of pose: Relaxes the body and begins to prepare it for corpse pose and deep relaxation. Releases the tension in the hips and in the legs.

Tips and Modifications: If you are going to perform this pose sitting, you can use a bolster or blanket to put under your sitting bones to help relax and to support the back. You can also use a bolster or blanket under the small of the back.

Corpse Pose

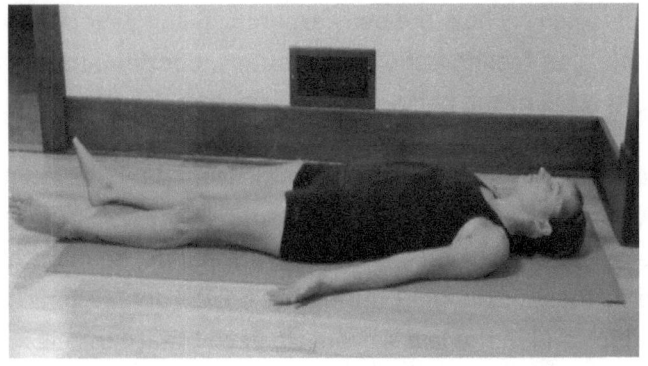

Posture: Begin on your back. Extend the legs out along the floor and the arms along the floor to your sides. Let the feet open gently and adjust your hips and shoulders to feel relaxed. Inhale and begin to relax each of the parts of the body. Exhale and focus on each muscle relaxing and of letting the tension that is in your body be released.

Focus of Pose: This pose is designed to enhance relaxation and for you to be aware of the process of relaxing each part of your body. Start with the toes and be mindful of each part of the body as you begin to relax them and release the tension and stress that is being held in the body. Release that tension into the mat and let your body feel open and light during each breath in the pose.

Length of Pose: 10-12 breaths

Benefits of pose: Relaxes the body and soothes the muscles to help your body feel light and open as you release the tension and stress that is captive in the body.

Tips and Modifications: Try to focus only on your breathing. Try to quiet the mind and bring the focus to each breath as you are relaxing in the pose. You may use a bolster or blanket under the knees, head and small of the back.

Salutation Seal Pose

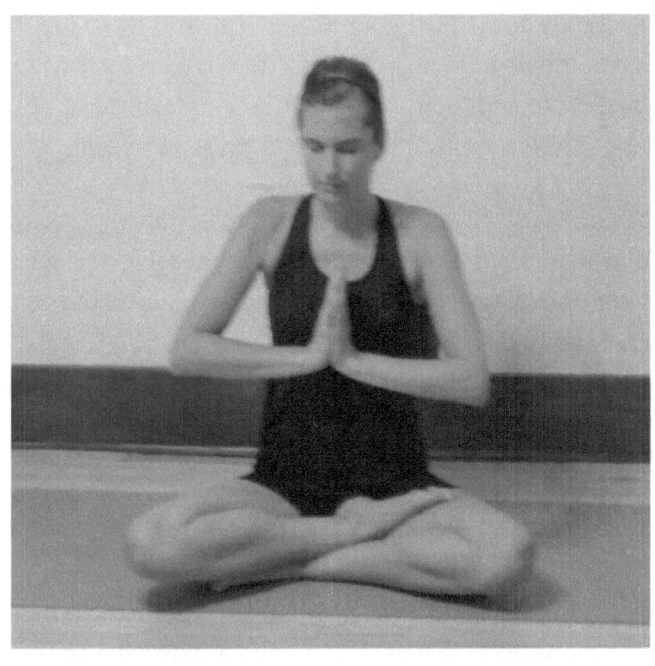

Posture: Begin in simple cross legged pose. You can cross the legs and either have the feet on the thighs, or on the floor. Let your hands rest lightly on the knees with the palms up. Keep the back straight and chest open. Keep the eyes closed. Inhale and bring both arms overhead. Exhale and release. Do this twice and then inhale to bring both arms forward, exhale to open the arms, squeezing the shoulders. Inhale and bring the arms forward, exhale and bring the hands together at the chest.

Focus of Pose: Use this pose to focus on the relaxation that you have created and the energy that you feel in the body.

Length of Pose: 10-12 breaths

Benefits of pose: Begin to focus on the breath and quiet the busy mind. Thank yourself for doing something positive for you, and continue to feel the relaxation through the body and focus on each breath during the pose.

Tips and Modifications: If it is uncomfortable for you to sit with your legs crossed, you may stretch them out along the ground and bend the knees slightly. You can also use a bolster or blanket to sit on to support the back muscles.

Meditation Basics

and Practice

One of the most challenging concepts of yoga to learn is meditation. For many people, being able to completely shut off the mind and find a place of peace and calm is difficult. It is challenging to shut off the noise, stress, thinking patterns and tension that usually are present when we sit down to relax.

You may not be able to master the art of meditation right away, but if you keep practicing and find your own methods, you will be able to quiet the mind.

Tips for meditation:

- Find a comfortable and quiet place
- Try to find a time when you are alone
- Find a comfortable position to sit in
- Try out a couple of different positions of sitting to see which one feels the best
- If you have trouble concentrating, try lighting a candle and keep your stare on the candle
- Try repeating a phrase or sound to help center yourself
- Chanting Om is a common way to send the sound vibrations through the body and calm the mind
- Try to keep the mind clear and focus only on your breathing

It is important to remember that you may not be able to sit down and center yourself right away. Learning how to really become still and present takes practice and time. Do not get disappointed if you are not able to become as relaxed as you would like, it will improve when you practice.

While everyone enjoys different kinds of sounds or phrases to practice during meditation, you may discover that you simply like to listen to soft music, or chimes. Chimes and singing bowls are a traditional way to relax and begin meditation and you can find the items that you need online.

You can also try a number of different meditation recordings that can help walk you through the beginning of your meditation and help you to focus on your breathing. It is important to find a certain kind of meditation that you can connect with and want to continue with.

The common poses or postures that you want to try and practice while learning meditation include salutation seal, simple cross legged pose or any seated position that you can stay in for a while and be comfortable. You may want to get a cushion or blanket to use as a prop underneath of your sitting bones. These can help with aligning the spine and allowing you to maintain correct posture.

There are a couple of meditations that you may want to begin with to help you get started.

Find Your Inner Calm:

As you sit in meditation, draw on three areas to focus on.
One, focus on what areas you can improve in your life.
Two, focus on what areas you need to improve in your life.
Three, focus on achieving them.
If we believe and see what we want to change, we can.

Positive Energy Meditation:

As you sit in meditation, begin to think about someone you love. As you think about that person, send them love and success. Next, think about someone that you are indifferent with such as a neighbor or co-worker, and send them love and success. Lastly, think about someone that you dislike and send them love and success. You will probably notice that it takes longer to send someone that you do not like the good energy, but if you practice this, you will learn to accept everyone for what they are and find it in you to love everyone.

Once you are able to wish love and happiness to all of the people in your life, you are open to receiving love and happiness.

Guided Relaxation:

- Begin in a reclined position on your back. Take a few moments to start to relax the entire body. Focus on any parts of the body that are sore or tight, and try to use each breath to relax them.
- Try to focus only on your breath.
- Take both hands and place them on the belly. Feel the breath start in the belly.
- Let the belly fill the hands each time that you inhale, and let the belly empty each time you exhale.
- Continue to feel the gentle rise and fall of the belly in your hands. Do this for a few breaths.
- Keep one hand on the belly and take the other hand up to the chest.
- Imagine the breath as a wave as it travels up from the belly, to the chest and out the nose. Do this for a few breaths.
- Keep one hand on the chest and take the other hand up to the forehead. Continue to feel the rise and fall of the belly and the chest as you let the touch of the hand on the forehead relax the eyes and relieve any tension between the eyes.
- Let the arms fall open to the sides along the ground.
- Continue to relax the entire body.
- Relax each of the toes. Relax up through the feet. Relax the legs. Relax the hips. Relax the belly and

the chest. Relax the shoulders.

- Relax the arms and through each hand and finger.
- Relax up through the neck. Relax the muscles in the face and relax the eyes.
- Let the body feel light and open each time that you inhale and let the weight of the body and the stress and tension sink into the floor each time you exhale.
- Inhale and on the exhale begin to sit up. When you are ready, return to a simple cross legged pose. Keep the back straight, the shoulders back, the chest open and the eyes closed.
- Inhale and bring the arms overhead, exhale the arms down. Repeat one more time.
- Inhale and bring the arms out in front, exhale open the arms. Inhale and bring the arms out in front, exhale and bring the hands together, and bring both hands to the chest.
- Continue to breathe and relax the body as you thank yourself for doing a great job.

Yoga for Aging

Yoga is not only a practice for young and healthy adults. Yoga reaches across all age groups and ability levels. When you begin a yoga practice at any age, you are able to see and learn more about yourself, your body and your abilities.

There are certain things that we cannot change, such as our age. There are certain things that we can change about the way we age. Accepting that our bodies change as we get older is one of the difficult parts of aging. We long to be the young and fit people that we once were, but suddenly may feel trapped in an older body.

The key to unlocking potential at any age is to move beyond the age limitations, and discover that we are very capable to learning and growing at any age. Yoga can help us accept who we are and what we are capable of, no matter what that may be.

You will read about some of the elderly students who have started a yoga practice later in life, and the ways that it has helped them to create a new perception of how much they are still able to do, and the remarkable ways that yoga has touched their lives and improved their well-being.

Many of the first responses to an older adult regarding a yoga practice include the "I am too old" way of thinking. But once you really open up to trying new things, you may pleasantly awe yourself and all that you are actually capable to do.

Our minds and ideas limit us to what we are willing to try and able to do. Yoga helps to open up our hearts and provides a positive and healthy way to keep improving wellness at any age.

Each of the students that are represented in this section are in a senior living facility. They range in age from 60-85. Each of them have a different reason for trying yoga and each has a different set of abilities.

The names have been changed, but their stories are true.

Meet Lara. Lara is 60 and has been diagnosed with Huntington's disease. She has some difficulty in moving her body and with uncontrollable spasms and tics that occur. She is determined to prolong any further effects of her illness, and do her best to retain the movement and ability that she has.

Lara was once a very active woman who aims to stay as active as she can. While her disease does create some limitations on what she is able to do, she finds that the gentle movements of yoga allow her to build strength, increase her mobility and relax.

Lara has been able to improve some of her physical and mental conditions by doing yoga every week in the facility where she lives. The yoga movements allow her to focus on deep breathing, relaxing and mental awareness to try and stop the decline of her mental facilities.

She is an inspiration to everyone who has been diagnosed with this disease and continues to stay as active as she can to prolong any further progression of the disease.

Meet Clara. Clara is 78 and has knee problems. She has lost a lot of her mobility because of her painful knees and was looking for a way to help regain some of the mobility that she once enjoyed.

Clara is not able to do many other forms of exercise, but has found that yoga helps her to connect with herself, take time for herself and to socialize with others. The mental benefits that Clara has seen with yoga inspire her to continue with her practice.

Clara is able to do most of the yoga exercises that are in the routine in this book, and makes modifications as needed to adjust to her body. She has learned to better accept her body and the abilities that she has. Though her knees are still painful for her, she does feel some relief from the yoga practice in the facility where she lives. She also has found friendship with some of her fellow students who also reside near her.

Meet Jane. Jane is 83 and has a tremor. She has also been recently diagnosed with Parkinson's disease. Her tremor has been a part of her life for many years, and has progressed since she has gotten older. The tremor is mainly in her right arm and causes her a lot of discomfort. It also makes it difficult for her to relax and feel comfortable at many of the daily tasks she does.

Jane began doing yoga because she was interested to see if it would help with her tremor, and as a way to still stay active. Jane was apprehensive at first to try yoga because it was something very new to her, and she was unsure if she would be able to do it.

Once she began her practice, she quickly adapted to the poses, gained some flexibility and felt good about herself for trying something new and making a positive step towards improving her symptoms.

Jane was recently diagnosed with Parkinson's disease and was recommended by her doctor to continue a yoga practice because it is one of the most beneficial and gentle ways to stay active and healthy.

Jane continues to enjoy the social aspects as well as the healthy benefits she is able to see during and after each yoga class.

Meet Doris. Doris is 84 and has a hip problem. Her hips cause her pain and discomfort, which makes some other forms of exercise difficult. Doris was interested in trying yoga because she wanted to see if it would help her regain some of the flexibility that she once had. Her hips had created difficulties for her and caused her to lose some of the range of motion that she needs.

Doris discovered that yoga not only helped to ease the pain associated with her hips, it also helped her to relax and quiet her mind. She is particularly fond of the relaxation sequence done at the end of practice, and finds that she is able to really focus on being present and not thinking or worrying about daily struggles.

Meet Grace. Grace is 82 and has Parkinson's disease. She has noticed the disease begin to create more challenges for her through speech and movement. She has uncontrollable spasms and movements often, and has a difficult time trying to remain still or to stop the spasms and movements.

She was once a very active woman who enjoyed sports and exercise. She is still very flexible and continues to inspire the yoga class members with her ability to stretch further than average.

She uses yoga to help her keep the strength that she needs in her muscles, and to help keep the flexibility to keep her active. Through yoga, she has found that she is able to relax her mind and her body enough to help her feel more at ease. Yoga is also recommended to her as a way to help curb the negative symptoms associated with her disease, and to help slow the decline of the symptoms. Doris has fully engaged with the class, and has also made more friends who accept her disease, and allow her to feel comfortable.

Mary is 76 and started taking yoga because she wanted to find a form of exercise that is gentle and will not bother her joints. She also wants to regain some of the flexibility that she used to have when she was younger. Through yoga practice, Mary has become more positive about herself, gained friendships and found a way to get exercise that is gentle but effective.

Mary also enjoys the relaxation that allows her to focus on breathing and calming the mind. Mary, like many of the other ladies, finds that yoga reminds her to not give up on being healthy and that she is young enough to feel good and keep exercising.

All of the ladies that take the senior yoga class share the common bond that they once were caretakers in their families. They were the wives and mothers who spend all o their time looking after their families, and did not have the time to spend on themselves.

Yoga for them is a way to finally take the time to focus on their health and do the things that they want to do. They also realized that they are not ready to be idle and do nothing about their health; they are ready to be active and try new things.

Yoga for Addiction Recovery

When you go through treatment, there are a number of emotions that you have to deal with, some for the first time in years. Through developing a healthy practice, such as Yoga, you can learn to deal with those emotions in a healthy way instead of with the old habits.

For most of us who have struggled with addiction of any kind, there were a lot of emotions that we did not deal with before because we hid behind the façade of a bottle or pill. When we no longer have our vices to lean on, we need to find something that will help us move on and pull ourselves out of the hole that we have dug.

I believe that the Yoga practice that you can learn from this book, and any additional resources that you use, can really help you to define a healthy role in your life, you have been called an addict, a loser and many other negative names, we all have and instead of dwelling on those, why not be called a Yogi? Or a success story? Sobriety can be challenging, and you can equip yourself with the tools that you need to help start a healthier lifestyle.

Don't give up on yourself, even if you feel as though everyone has given up on you, believe that you are strong enough to do this, and that you will do it. I know I am more than a recovering alcoholic, or as I like to say "sobriety challenged" and you need to know that you are too.

If you are going through any kind of addiction recovery,

there are some focus areas that you can work on during each routine. Some of the main areas that you want to focus on while performing the poses in this book include:

- As you begin to relax the mind and center yourself for your practice, begin to focus on the now and now the past. Let the painful addictions go, and breathe in new breath for sobriety.

- As you twist into the pose, take the time to gaze softly over the shoulders and reflect on what is behind you and be willing to move forward as you turn back to the front.

- **The** flexibility of the spine reminds us that we are strong, subtle and full of motion to improve not only our flexibility, but also our wellness.

- Balancing the body is key to regaining strength. The more that you focus on creating a new and healthy balance in the pose, you can extend through the stretch and create a more balanced you.

- Reflect on the relaxation that you are feeling, but the warmth of the body that you are feeling from movement and the stretches. Let yourself go deeper into the stretch with each exhale and enjoy the relaxation.

- Completely open up on each side of the stretch and

begin to allow yourself and your true self to be seen and exposed, while you build strength and endurance each time that you practice the pose.

- Each day of sobriety requires you to be flexible and create balance. This pose teaches you to continue to strive for more balance and more flexibility.

- Begin each pose as you do each day in sobriety with the ability to stretch, improve and listen to your own body.

- Balance is difficult to maintain when you are beginning sobriety, but the more that you practice and the more that you believe that you can do it, you will be able to.

- Becoming more flexible can help you regain the strength that you need for your sobriety. Letting yourself go further into the stretch and listening to your breath can help you become stronger.

- These poses inhibit strength and portray a warrior that is strong and flexible. Think of yourself on a mountain top while you look over your past, and create a strong presence towards your sobriety and goals.

- We keep a lot of tension and stress in the hip areas. By opening up the hips and stretching them, you may find that you release stress and negative energy that have been piling up. Allow yourself to free that stress and tension and look forward to the new beginnings with openness.

- Focus on pushing the weight of the problems that addiction has caused behind you, and focus on reaching up to the new goals that you have.

- Focus on the strength in each pose and how you are looking forward to everything that sobriety can bring for you and be open and strong to accept it.

- Look up at what you are able to do and build on the strength that you already have to reach up towards sobriety.

- Balancing yourself in these poses can help you realize the balance that you are creating in your life and the stronger that you get, the more you will be able to hold yourself strong.

References:

Index of Asanas, Yoga Journal,
http://www.yogajournal.com/poses/finder/browse_index

Yoga History, American Yoga Association,
http://www.americanyogaassociation.org/general.html

Benefits of Yoga, Yoga Movement,
http://www.yogamovement.com/resources/benefits.html

Meditation Basics, Meditation Techniques,
http://www.meditationsutras.com/

About the Author

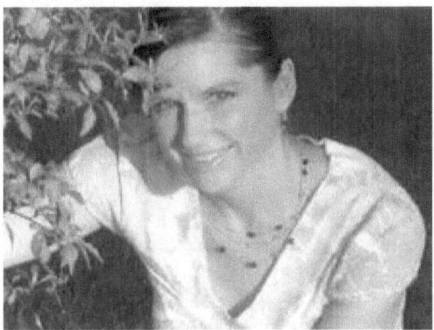

Kristi Abbott, owner of BodySava Yoga and Reflexology lives in Fargo, ND. She has been practicing and teaching yoga for over a decade and has initiated a yoga movement in her area to reach out to those in recovery and teaches at a treatment facility to groups of students who are working towards becoming sober. She also works with the elderly to teach yoga.

Contact the Author:

bodysava@gmail.com

www.bodysava.com

www.ingramcontent.com/pod-product-compliance
Lightning Source LLC
Chambersburg PA
CBHW031247280526
45784CB00004B/1755